KETO CH

RECII

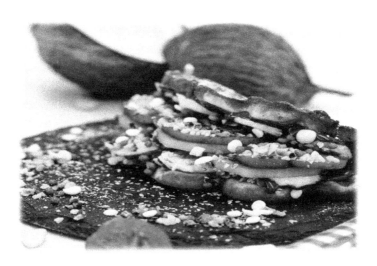

Eat Delicious Treats and Stay in Ketosis with This Mouth-Watering Low-Carb Waffle Recipes That Will Satisfy Your Sugar Cravings

Megan Slim

TABLE OF CONTENT

© Copyright 2020 by Megan Slim -- All rights reserved.

The information in the following pages is broadly considered a truthful and accurate account of facts and as such, any inattention, use, or misuse of the information in question by the reader will render any resulting actions solely under their purview. There are no scenarios in which the publisher or the original author of this work can be in any fashion deemed liable for any hardship or damages that may befall them after undertaking information described herein.

Additionally, the information in the following pages is intended only for informational purposes and should thus be thought of as universal. As befitting its nature, it is presented without assurance regarding its prolonged validity or interim quality. Trademarks that are mentioned are done without written consent and can in no way be considered an endorsement from the trademark holder.

Tips & Tricks to Make Amazing Chaffles

Gluten-free chaffles combine two of America's most popular foods, cheese, and waffles, and they appear everywhere on social media. They are the undisputed stars of many Pinterest forums and Instagram stories, and I've also found several recipe groups on Facebook with tens of thousands of members. Join one of them, and you'll be bombarded with an endless stream of gorgeous photos - and yes, most of them look truly delightful. While this concept is new to some of you, this overwhelming trend seems to have emerged across America. It occurs mainly in eaters on a limited diet. Really, who can blame them, the ketogenic diet lovers love to substitute for a low-carb, cheap, easy-to-make, completely grain-free bread.

Ready to jump to the bar? Basic chaffles only require a few daily ingredients—eggs and a handful of grated cheese with a little baking soda if desired to make it very light. Then you are limited only by your imagination and personal taste.

I personally prefer chaffle recipes that contain coconut or almond flour for a less moist taste (you can only use protein for the same effect). Extraordinary bread is even less spicy.

Use mayonnaise as a binder, and it really tastes like soft white bread and pillow. Sweet spots are topped with cream cheese. Optional additions give special notes—for example, cocoa powder, vanilla, chocolate chips, and/or cinnamon as a dessert of turkey or meat slices, jalapeño slices, herbal spices, or more seasoned garlic spices.

You can double up on the recipe below to make super tasty waffles (waffles are waffles, right?). But when you use it for sandwiches, the size of a mini waffle maker is perfect. Here are some tips for making perfect recipes: Preheat the waffle iron for a few minutes before using it and bring it to temperature.

Even if your waffle iron is brand new and has a whole Teflon coating, lightly spray the iron with cooking spray or melt the melted butter in all corners before adding the batter. Otherwise, the chaffles can jam.

Fill the hot iron with a light hand. The dough will come off after closing the lid, and if you mix it with the waffles, the dough will come out, leaving a terrible mess. Be patient. Resist the urge to open the waffle iron while you're cooking.

If you're serving more than one serving, keep the grill hot and crisp in the oven at 200 degrees. Don't be afraid to be creative. Try different types of cheese, herbs, food supplements, and side dishes.

Do not check for soot or burning signs by opening the waffle iron too quickly! You want it to cook until ripe and crunchy. If nothing else, stretch the cooking side a little more than you think. You can certainly experiment with other cheeses that are good for keto — goat cheese and halloumi work well — but mozzarella is usually recommended because it's mild and not as high as other choices.

 If you want more protein and flavor, you can also add one slice of ham when mixing egg and cheese. Bacon can work, too (enough if you're on a strict keto diet). If you prefer sweet cubes, substitute the mozzarella cream. I like this tip! I can't imagine mozzarella on my cakes. Sprinkle some extra cheese on the waffle iron before adding the egg and cheese mixture to get a warm, crispy crust.

It may be difficult to make it super crunchy on your plate because the steam from the stew softens them like all waves. It is best to eat or freeze them immediately, although I have found that a little almond flour helps the texture.

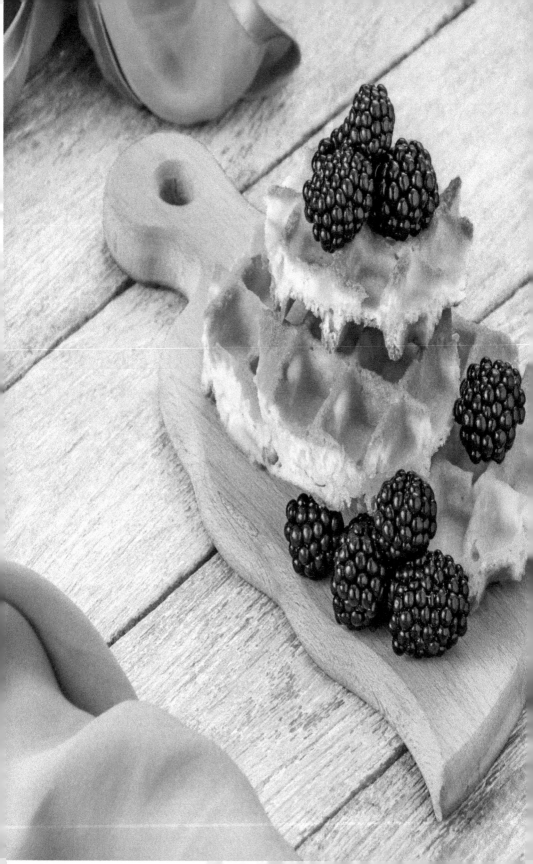

1.Jalapeno Chaffle

✕ **Servings**: 2

🥄 **Preparation Time**: 5 Minutes

⏰ **Cooking Time**: 10 Minutes

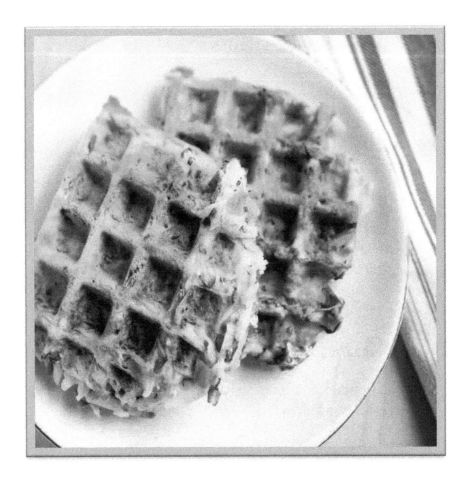

📋 *Ingredients* :

- ❖ 2 eggs, whisked

- ❖ 2 cups almond milk

- ❖ 2 tablespoons avocado oil

- ❖ ½ cup cheddar, shredded

- ❖ 1 cup almond flour

- ❖ 1 tablespoon baking powder

- ❖ A pinch of salt and black pepper

- ❖ ½ teaspoon garlic powder

- ❖ 2 Jalapenos, minced

Directions:

1. In a bowl, mix the eggs with the milk, oil, and the other ingredients and whisk well.

2. Preheat the waffle iron, pour 1/6 of the batter, cook for

8 minutes and transfer to a plate.

3. Repeat with the rest of the batter and serve.

Nutrition: Calories: 381; Fat: 14g; Fiber: 3.6g;

Carbs: 13g; Protein: 13g

2.Green Chili Chaffle

✗ **Servings**: 2

🥄 **Preparation Time**: 10 Minutes

⏰ **Cooking Time**: 10 Minutes

📋 *Ingredients* :

- ❖ 2 eggs, whisked

- ❖ 1 and ½ cup almond flour

- ❖ ½ cup cream cheese, soft

- ❖ ½ cup almond milk

- ❖ 1 teaspoon baking soda

- ❖ A pinch of salt and black k pepper

- ❖ ½ cup green chilies, minced

- ❖ 1 tablespoon chives, chopped

Directions:

1. In a bowl, mix the eggs with the flour, cream cheese, and the other ingredients and whisk.

2. Preheat the waffle iron, pour 1/6 of the batter, close the waffle maker, cook for 8 minutes and transfer to a plate.

3. Repeat with the rest of the batter and serve.

Nutrition: Calories: 265; Fat: 7; Fiber: 3 Carbs: 5.4;

Protein: 6

3.Hot Pork Chaffles

✕ **Servings**: 2

🥄 **Preparation Time**: 10 Minutes

⏰ **Cooking Time**: 10 Minutes

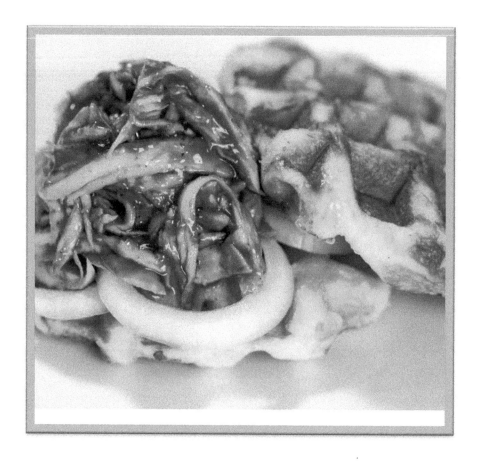

📋 Ingredients :

- ❖ 1 cup pulled pork, cooked

- ❖ 2 tablespoons parmesan, grated

- ❖ 2 eggs, whisked

- ❖ 2 red chilies, minced

- ❖ 1 cup almond milk

- ❖ 1 cup almond flour

- ❖ 2 tablespoons coconut oil, melted

- ❖ 1 teaspoon baking powder

Directions:

1. In a bowl, mix the pulled pork with the eggs, parmesan, and the other ingredients and whisk well.

2. Heat up the waffle maker, pour ¼ of the chaffle mix, cook for 8 minutes and transfer to a plate.

3. Repeat with the rest of the mix and serve.

Nutrition: Calories: 300; **Fat:** 13g; **Fiber:** 4g **Carbs:** 7.2g; Protein: 15g

4.Spicy Chicken Chaffles

🍴 **Servings**: 2

🥄 **Preparation Time**: 10 Minutes

⏰ **Cooking Time**: 10 Minutes

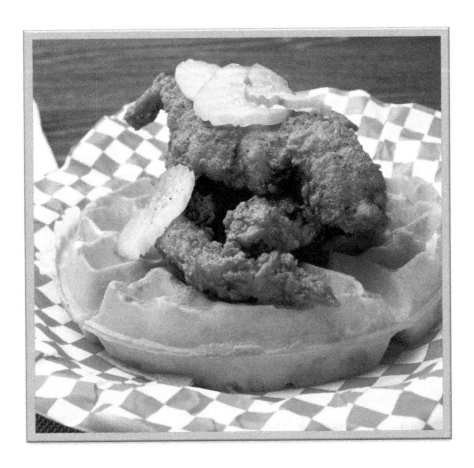

📋 *Ingredients*:

- ❖ 2 eggs, whisked
- ❖ 1 cup rotisserie chicken, skinless, boneless, and shredded
- ❖ 1 cup mozzarella, shredded
- ❖ ½ cup milk
- ❖ 2 teaspoons chili powder
- ❖ 1 teaspoon sriracha sauce
- ❖ 1 tablespoon chives, chopped
- ❖ ½ teaspoon baking powder

Directions:

1. In a bowl, mix the eggs with the chicken, mozzarella, and the other ingredients and whisk.

2. Preheat the waffle maker, pour ¼ of the batter, cook for 10 minutes, and transfer to a plate.

3. Repeat with the rest of the batter and serve.

Nutrition: Calories: 320; Fat: 8g; Fiber: 2g Carbs: 5.3g; Protein: 12g

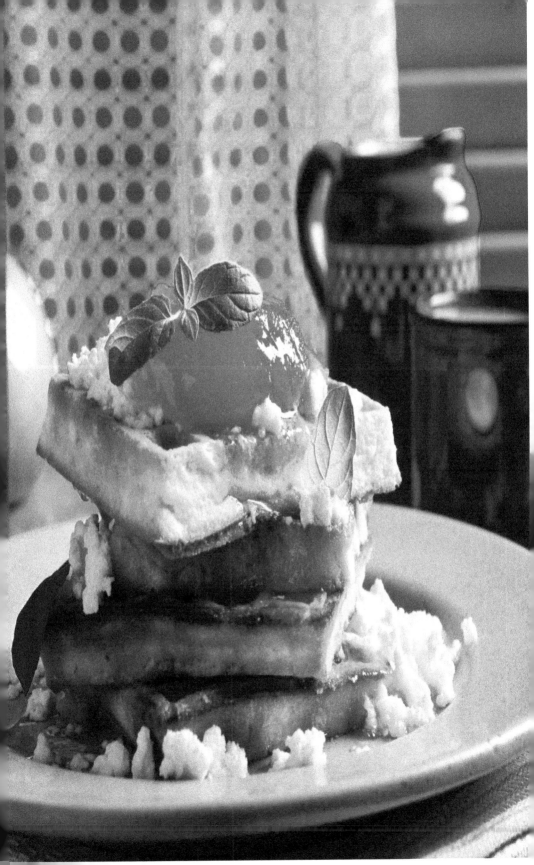

5.Spicy Ricotta Chaffles

Servings: 2

Preparation Time: 10 Minutes

Cooking Time: 10 Minutes

Ingredients:

- ❖ 2 cups coconut flour

- ❖ 1 and ½ cups coconut milk

- ❖ 2 tablespoons olive oil

- ❖ A pinch of salt and black pepper

- ❖ ½ cup ricotta cheese

- ❖ 1 teaspoon baking powder

- ❖ 2 eggs, whisked

- ❖ ½ cup chives, chopped

- ❖ 1 Red chili pepper, minced

❖ 1 Jalapeno, chopped

Directions:

1. In a bowl, mix the flour with the milk, oil, and the other ingredients and whisk well.

2. Heat up the waffle iron, pour ¼ of the batter, cook for 10 minutes and transfer to a plate.

3. Repeat with the rest of the chaffle mix and serve.

Nutrition: Calories: 262; Fat: 8g; Fiber: 2.4g;

Carbs: 3.2g; Protein: 8g

6.Double Decker Chaffle

X **Servings**: 2

🥄 **Preparation Time**: 7 Minutes

⏰ **Cooking Time**: 10 Minutes

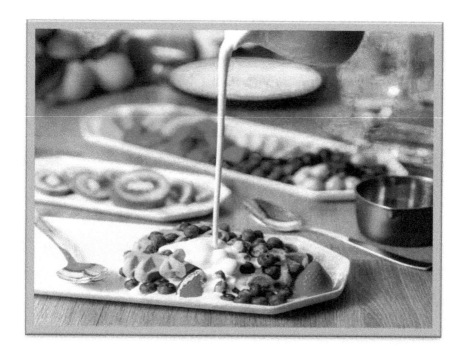

📋 Ingredients :

❖ 1 Large egg

❖ 1 cup shredded cheese

Topping:

- ❖ 1 Keto chocolate ball

- ❖ 2 oz. Cranberries

- ❖ 2 oz. Blueberries

- ❖ 4 oz. Cranberries puree

Directions:

1. Make 2 minutes dash waffles.

2. Put cranberries and blueberries in the freezer for about hours.

3. For serving, arrange keto chocolate balls between the chaffles.

4. Top with frozen berries,

5. Serve and enjoy!

Nutrition: **Protein**: 78; **Fat**: 223; **Carbohydrates**: 31

7.Cinnamon and Vanilla Chaffle

✗ **Servings**: 2

🥄 **Preparation Time**: 5 Minutes

⏰ **Cooking Time**: 7-9 Minutes

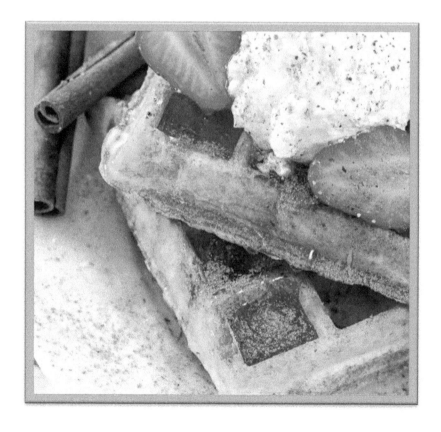

📋 **Ingredients :**

Batter:

- ❖ 4 eggs

- ❖ 4 Ounces sour cream

- ❖ 1 teaspoon vanilla extract

- ❖ 1 teaspoon cinnamon

- ❖ ¼ cup stevia

- ❖ 5 tablespoons coconut flour

Other:

- ❖ 2 tablespoons coconut oil to brush the waffle maker

- ❖ ½ teaspoon cinnamon for garnishing the chaffles

Directions:

1. Preheat the waffle maker.

2. Add the eggs and sour cream to a bowl and stir with a wire whisk until just combined.

3. Add the vanilla extract, cinnamon, and Stevia and mix until combined.

4. Stir in the coconut flour and stir until combined.

5. Brush the heated waffle maker with coconut oil and add a few tablespoons of the batter.

6. Cover and cook for about 7–8 minutes, depending on your waffle maker.

7. Serve and enjoy.

Nutrition: Calories: 224; Fat: 11g; **Carbs:** 8.4g;

Sugar: 0.5; **Protein:** 7.7g; **Sodium:** 77mg

8.Chaffles and Ice-cream Platter

✖ **Servings**: 2

🥄 **Preparation Time**: 10 Minutes

⏰ **Cooking Time**: 5 Minutes

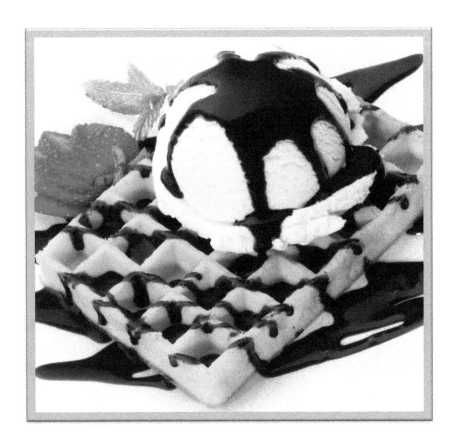

🗒 Ingredients :

- ❖ 2 Keto brownie chaffles

- ❖ 2 Scoops vanilla keto ice cream

- ❖ 8 oz. Strawberries, sliced

- ❖ Keto chocolate sauce

Directions:

1. Arrange chaffles, ice cream, strawberries slice in serving plate.

2. Drizzle chocolate sauce on top.

3. Serve and enjoy!

Nutrition: Protein: 26%; Fat: 68%; Carbohydrates: 6%

9.Choco Chip Pumpkin Chaffle

✗ **Servings**: 2

🥄 **Preparation Time**: 10 Minutes

⏰ **Cooking Time**: 15 Minutes

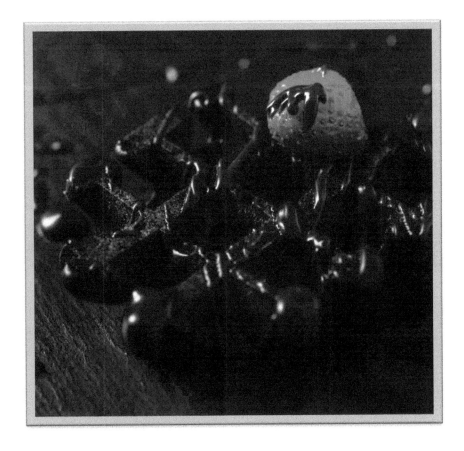

Ingredients:

- ❖ 1 egg, lightly beaten

- ❖ 1 tablespoon almond flour

- ❖ 1 tablespoon unsweetened chocolate chips

- ❖ 1/4 teaspoon pumpkin pie spice

- ❖ 2 tablespoons Swerve

- ❖ 1 tablespoon pumpkin puree

- ❖ 1/2 cup mozzarella cheese, shredded

Directions:

1. Preheat your waffle maker.

2. In a small bowl, mix egg and pumpkin puree.

3. Add pumpkin pie spice, Swerve, almond flour, and cheese and mix well.

4. Stir in chocolate chips.

5. Spray waffle maker with cooking spray.

6. Introduce half batter in the hot waffle maker and cook for 4 minutes. Repeat with the remaining batter.

7. Serve and enjoy.

Nutrition: Calories: 130; Fat: 9.2;

Carbohydrates: 5.9; **Sugar**: 0.6; **Protein**: 6.6

10. Sausage & Pepperoni Chaffle Sandwich

✄ **Servings:** 2

🥄 **Preparation Time:** 8 Minutes

⏰ **Cooking Time:** 10 Minutes

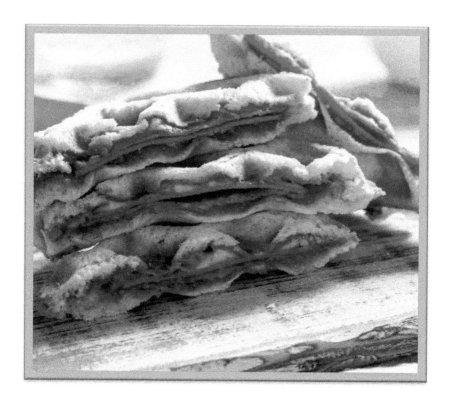

Ingredients :

❖ Cooking spray

❖ 2 Cervelat sausage, sliced into rounds

❖ 12 pieces pepperoni

❖ 6 mushroom slices

❖ 4 teaspoons mayonnaise

❖ 4 large white onion rings

❖ 4 basic chaffles

Directions:

1. Spray your skillet with oil.

2. Place over medium heat.

3. Cook sausage until both sides turn brown

4. Transfer on a plate.

5. Cook the pepperoni and mushrooms for 2 minutes.

6. Spread mayo on the top of the chaffle.

7. Top with the sausage, pepperoni, mushrooms, and onion rings.

8. Top with another chaffle.

Nutrition: Calories: 373; Total Fat: 24.4g; Saturated Fat: 6g; Cholesterol: 27mg; Sodium: 717mg; Potassium: 105mg; Total Carbohydrates: 28g; Dietary Fiber: 1.1g; Protein: 8.1g; Total Sugars: 4.5g

11. Blueberry Cream Cheese Chaffles

X **Servings**: 2

P **Preparation Time**: 10 Minutes

⏰ **Cooking Time**: 8 Minutes

Ingredients:

- ❖ 1 Organic egg, beaten
- ❖ 1 tablespoon cream cheese, softened
- ❖ 3 tablespoons almond flour
- ❖ 1/4 teaspoon organic baking powder
- ❖ 1 teaspoon organic blueberry extract
- ❖ 5-6 Fresh blueberries

Directions:

1. Preheat a mini waffle maker and then grease it.

2. In a bowl, place all the ingredients except blueberries and beat until well combined.

3. Fold in the blueberries.

4. Divide the mixture into five portions.

5. Place one portion of the mixture into the preheated waffle iron and cook for about 3-4 minutes or until golden brown.

6. Repeat with the remaining mixture.

7. Serve warm.

Nutrition: Calories: 120; Net Carbs: 1.8g; Fat: 9.6g; Saturated Fat: 2.2g; Carbohydrates: 3.1g; Dietary Fiber: 1.3g;   Sugar: 1g;   Protein:3.2g

12. Blackberry Chaffles

✖ **Servings**: 2

🥄 **Preparation Time**: 10 Minutes

⏰ **Cooking Time**: 8 Minutes

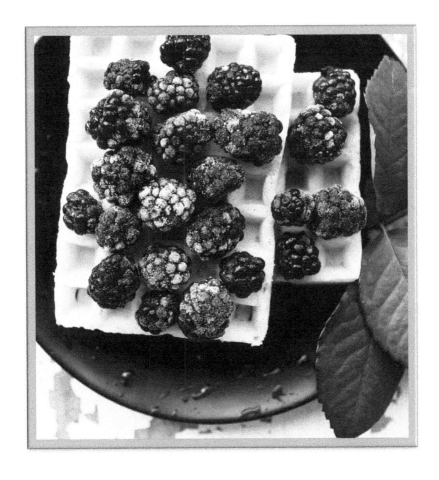

📋 Ingredients :

- ❖ 1 Organic egg, beaten
- ❖ 1/3 cup Mozzarella cheese, shredded
- ❖ 1 teaspoon cream cheese, softened
- ❖ 1 teaspoon coconut flour
- ❖ 1/4 teaspoon organic baking powder
- ❖ 3/4 teaspoon powdered Erythritol
- ❖ 1/4 teaspoon ground cinnamon
- ❖ 1/4 teaspoon organic vanilla extract
- ❖ A pinch of salt
- ❖ 1 tablespoon fresh blackberries

Directions:

1. Preheat a mini waffle maker and then grease it.

2. In a bowl, place all the ingredients except for blackberries and beat until well combined.

3. Fold in the blackberries.

4. Place half of the mixture into the preheated waffle iron and cook for about four minutes or until golden brown.

5. Repeat with the remaining mixture.

Nutrition: Calories: 121; **Net Carbs**: 2.7g;

Fat:7.5g; **Saturated Fat**: 3.3g; **Carbohydrates**: 4.5g;

Dietary Fiber: 1.8g; **Sugar**: 0.9g; **Protein**: 8.9g

13.   Strawberry Chaffles

✗ **Servings**: 2

🥄 **Preparation Time**: 10 Minutes

⏰ **Cooking Time**: 8 Minutes

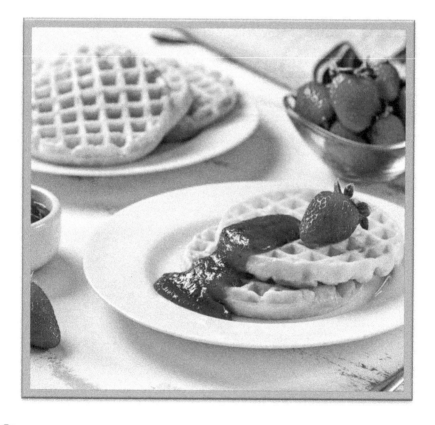

📋 # Ingredients :

❖ 1 organic egg, beaten

- ❖ ¼ cup Mozzarella cheese, shredded

- ❖ 1 tablespoon cream cheese, softened

- ❖ ¼ teaspoon organic baking powder

- ❖ 1 teaspoon organic strawberry extract

- ❖ 2 fresh strawberries, hulled and sliced

Directions:

1. Preheat a mini waffle maker and then grease it.

2. In a bowl, place all ingredients except strawberry slices and beat until well combined.

3. Fold in the strawberry slices.

4. Place half of the mixture into the preheated waffle iron and cook for about four minutes or until golden brown.

5. Repeat with the remaining mixture.

6. Serve warm.

Nutrition: Calories: 69; Net Carbs: 1.6g; Fat: 4.6g; Saturated Fat: 2.2g; Carbohydrates: 1.9g; Dietary Fiber: 0.3g; Sugar: 1g;   Protein: 4.2g

14. Raspberry Chaffles

🍴 **Servings**: 2

🥄 **Preparation Time**: 10 Minutes

⏰ **Cooking Time**: 8 Minutes

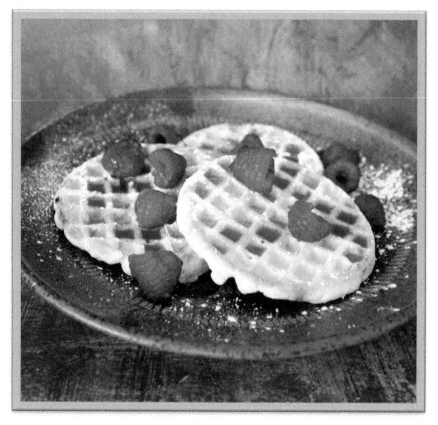

📋 *Ingredients:*

- ❖ 1 organic egg, beaten
- ❖ 1 tablespoon cream cheese, softened

- ❖ ½ cup Mozzarella cheese, shredded
- ❖ 1 tablespoon powdered Erythritol
- ❖ ¼ teaspoon organic raspberry extract
- ❖ ¼ teaspoon organic vanilla extract

Directions:

1. Preheat a mini waffle maker and then grease it.

2. In a medium bowl, place all ingredients, and with a fork, mix until well combined.

3. Place half of the mixture into the preheated waffle iron and cook for about four minutes or until golden brown.

4. Repeat with the remaining mixture.

5. Serve warm.

Nutrition: Calories: 69; **Net Carbs**: 0.6g; **Fat**: 5.2g;

Saturated Fat: 2.5g; **Carbohydrates**: 0.6g; **Dietary Fiber**: 00g;

Sugar: 0.2g; **Protein**: 5.6g

15.   2- Berries Chaffles

Servings: 2

Preparation Time: 10 Minutes

Cooking Time: 10 Minutes

Ingredients :

- ✓ 1 organic egg
- ✓ 1 teaspoon organic vanilla extract
- ✓ 1 tablespoon of almond flour
- ✓ 1 teaspoon organic baking powder
- ✓ A pinch of ground cinnamon
- ✓ 1 cup Mozzarella cheese, shredded
- ✓ 2 tablespoons fresh blueberries
- ✓ 2 tablespoons fresh blackberries

Directions:

1. Preheat a waffle maker and then grease it.

2. In a bowl, place the egg and vanilla extract and beat well.

3. Add the flour, baking powder, and cinnamon and mix well.

4. Add the Mozzarella cheese and mix until just combined.

5. Gently fold in the berries.

6. Place half of the mixture into the preheated waffle iron and cook for about 4-5 minutes or until golden brown.

7. Repeat with the remaining mixture.

8. Serve warm.

Nutrition: Calories: 112; Net Carbs: 3.8g; Fat: 6.7g; Saturated Fat: 2.3g; Carbohydrates: 5g; Dietary Fiber: 1.2g; Sugar: 1.9g; Protein: 7g

16. Italian Seasoning Chaffles

✕ **Servings**: 2

🥄 **Preparation Time**: 10 Minutes

⏰ **Cooking Time**: 8 Minutes

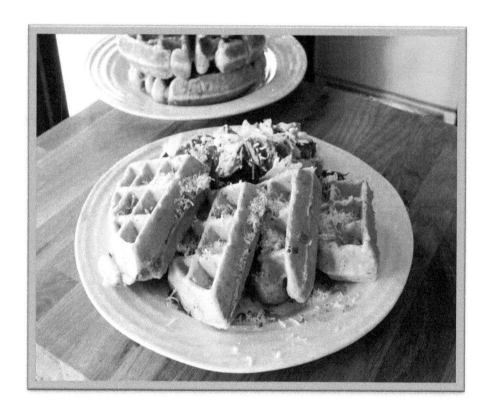

📋 **Ingredients :**

- ❖ ½ cup Mozzarella cheese, shredded
- ❖ 1 tablespoon Parmesan cheese, shredded
- ❖ 1 Organic egg
- ❖ ¾ teaspoon coconut flour
- ❖ ¼ teaspoon organic baking powder
- ❖ 1/8 teaspoon Italian seasoning
- ❖ A pinch of salt

Directions:

1. Preheat a mini waffle maker and then grease it.

2. In a medium bowl, place all ingredients, and with a fork, mix until well combined.

3. Place half of the mixture into the preheated waffle iron and cook for about 3-4 minutes or until golden brown.

4. Repeat with the remaining mixture.

5. Serve warm.

Nutrition: Calories: 86; **Net Carbs**: 1.9g; **Fat**: 5g;

Saturated Fat: 2.6g; **Carbohydrates**: 3.8g

Dietary Fiber: 1.9g; **Sugar:** 0.6g; **Protein:** 6.5g

17. Garlic Herb Blend Seasoning Chaffles

✖ **Servings**: 2

✒ **Preparation Time**: 10 Minutes

⏰ **Cooking Time**: 8 Minutes

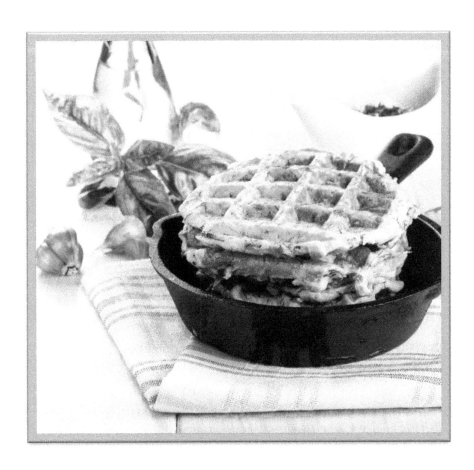

📋 **Ingredients :**

- ❖ 1 Large organic egg, beaten
- ❖ 1/4 cup Parmesan cheese, shredded
- ❖ 1/4 cup Mozzarella cheese, shredded
- ❖ 1/2 tablespoon butter, melted
- ❖ 1 teaspoon garlic herb blend seasoning
- ❖ Salt, to taste

Directions:

1. Preheat a mini waffle maker and then grease it.

2. In a bowl, place all the ingredients and beat until well combined.

3. Place half of the mixture into the preheated waffle iron and cook for about 3-4 minutes or until golden brown.

4. Repeat with the remaining mixture.

5. Serve warm.

Nutrition: Calories: 115; Net Carbs: 1.1g; Fat: 8.8g;

Saturated Fat: 4.7g; **Carbohydrates**: 1.2g; **Dietary Fiber**: 0.1g;

Sugar: 0.2g; **Protein:** 8g

18.   BBQ Rub Chaffles

🍴 **Servings**: 2

🥄 **Preparation Time**: 5 Minutes

⏰ **Cooking Time**: 20 Minutes

📋 Ingredients :

- ❖ 2 Organic eggs, beaten
- ❖ 1 cup Cheddar cheese, shredded
- ❖ ½ teaspoon BBQ rub
- ❖ ¼ teaspoon organic baking powder

Directions:

1. Preheat a mini waffle maker and then grease it.

2. In a medium bowl, place all ingredients, and with a fork, mix until well combined.

3. Place ¼ of the mixture into the preheated waffle iron and cook for about 5 minutes or until golden brown.

4. Repeat with the remaining mixture.

5. Serve warm.

Nutrition: Calories: 146; Net Carbs: 0.7g; Fat: 11.6g; Saturated Fat: 6.6g; Carbohydrates: 0.7g; Dietary Fiber: 0g; Sugar: 0.3g; Protein: 9.8g

19.   Bagel Seasoning Chaffles

✗   **Servings:** 2

✎   **Preparation Time:** 10 Minutes

⏰   **Cooking Time:** 20 Minutes

📋   **Ingredients** :

- ❖ 1 Large organic egg
- ❖ 1 cup Mozzarella cheese, shredded
- ❖ 1 tablespoon almond flour

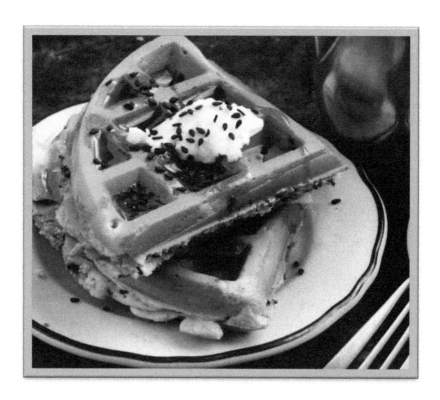

- ❖ 1 teaspoon organic baking powder
- ❖ 2 teaspoons bagel seasoning
- ❖ ¼ teaspoon garlic powder
- ❖ ¼ teaspoon onion powder

Directions:

1. Preheat a mini waffle maker and then grease it.

2. In a medium bowl, place all ingredients, and with a fork, mix until well combined.

3. Place ¼ of the mixture into the preheated waffle iron and cook for about 3-4 minutes or until golden brown.

4. Repeat with the remaining mixture.

5. Serve warm.

Nutrition: Calories: 73; **Net Carbs:** 2g; **Fat:** 5.5g;

Saturated Fat: 1.5g; **Carbohydrates:** 2.3g

Dietary Fiber: 0.3g; **Sugar:** 0.9g; **Protein:** 3.7g

20. Rosemary Chaffles

✖ **Servings**: 2

✎ **Preparation Time**: 5 Minutes

⏰ **Cooking Time**: 8 Minutes

📋 *Ingredients*:

- ❖ 1 Organic egg, beaten

- ❖ ½ cup Cheddar cheese, shredded

- ❖ 1 tablespoon almond flour

- ❖ 1 tablespoon fresh rosemary, chopped

- ❖ A pinch of salt and freshly ground black pepper

Directions:

1. Preheat a mini waffle maker and then grease it.

2. For the chaffles, in a medium bowl, place all ingredients and with a fork, mix until well combined.

3. Place half of the mixture into the preheated waffle iron

and cook for about 3-4 minutes or until golden brown.

4. Repeat with the remaining mixture.

5. Serve warm.

Nutrition: Calories: 173; **Net Carbs**: 1.1g; **Fat**: 13.7g; Saturated Fat: 6.9g; **Carbohydrates**: 2.2g; **Dietary Fiber**: 1.1g; Sugar: 0.4g; **Protein**: 9.9g

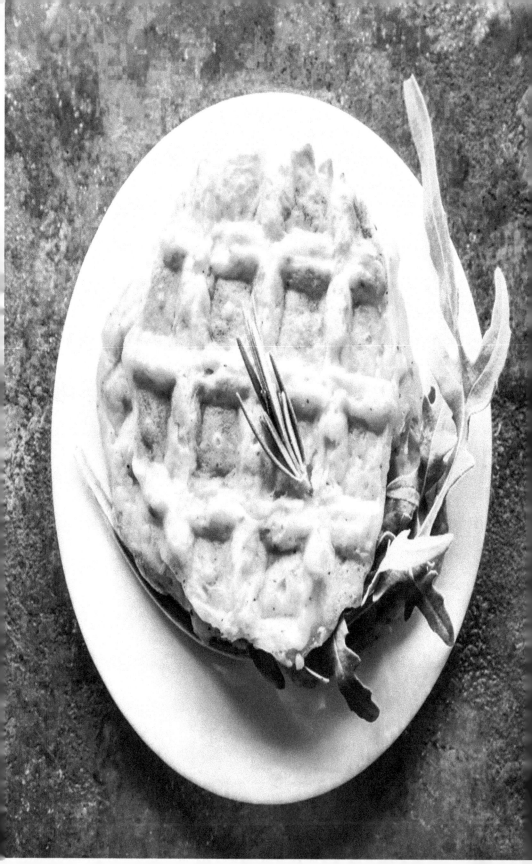

21. Salmon & Cheese Sandwich Chaffles

🍴 **Servings**: 2

🥄 **Preparation Time**: 15 Minutes

⏰ **Cooking Time**: 24 Minutes

📋 ## Ingredients :

For the Chaffles:

- ❖ 2 Organic eggs
- ❖ ½ Ounce butter, melted
- ❖ 1 cup mozzarella cheese, shredded
- ❖ 2 tablespoons almond flour
- ❖ A pinch of salt

For the Filling:

- ❖ ½ cup smoked salmon
- ❖ 1/3 cup avocado, peeled, pitted, and sliced
- ❖ 2 tablespoons feta cheese, crumbled

Directions:

1. Preheat a mini waffle maker and then grease it.

2. For the chaffles, in a medium bowl, put all ingredients and with a fork, mix until well combined.

3. Place ¼ of the mixture into the preheated waffle iron and cook for about 5–6 minutes.

4. Repeat with the remaining mixture.

5. Serve each chaffle with the filling ingredients.

Nutrition: Calories: 169; Net Carbs: 1.2g

Total Fat: 13.5g; **Saturated Fat**: 5g; **Cholesterol**: 101mg;

Sodium: 319mg; **Total Carbs**: 2.8g; **Fiber**: 1.6g; **Sugar**: 0.6g;

Protein: 8.9g

22. Salmon & Cream Sandwich Chaffles

✕ **Servings**: 2

🥄 **Preparation Time**: 10 Minutes

⏰ **Cooking Time**: 8 Minutes

📋 Ingredients :

For the Chaffles:

- ❖ 1 Organic egg, beaten
- ❖ ½ cup cheddar cheese, shredded
- ❖ 1 tablespoon almond flour
- ❖ 1 tablespoon fresh rosemary, chopped

For the Filling:

- ❖ ¼ cup smoked salmon
- ❖ 1 teaspoon fresh dill, chopped
- ❖ 2 tablespoons cream

Directions:

1. Preheat a mini waffle maker and then grease it.

2. For the chaffles, in a medium bowl, put all ingredients and with a fork, mix until well combined.

3. Place half of the mixture into the preheated waffle iron and cook for about 3–4 minutes.

4. Repeat with the remaining mixture.

5. Serve each chaffle with the filling ingredients.

Nutrition: Calories: 202; **Net Carbs:** 1.7g

Total Fat: 15.1g; **Saturated Fat:** 7.5g

Cholesterol: 118mg; **Sodium:** 345mg

Total Carbs: 2.9g; **Fiber:** 1.2g; **Sugar:** 0.7g; **Protein:** 13.2g

23. **Tuna Sandwich Chaffles**

✕ **Servings**: 2

🥄 **Preparation Time**: 10 Minutes

⏰ **Cooking Time**: 8 Minutes

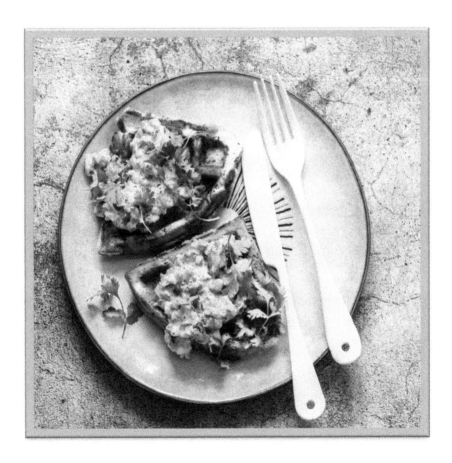

📋 Ingredients :

For the Chaffles:

- ❖ 1 Organic egg, beaten
- ❖ ½ cup cheddar cheese, shredded
- ❖ 1 tablespoon almond flour
- ❖ A pinch of salt

For the Filling:

- ❖ ¼ cup water-packed tuna, flaked
- ❖ 2 Lettuce leaves

Directions:

1. Preheat a mini waffle maker and then grease it.

2. For the chaffles, in a medium bowl, put all ingredients and with a fork, mix until well combined.

3. Place half of the mixture into the preheated waffle iron and cook for about 3–4 minutes.

4. Repeat with the remaining mixture.

5. Serve each chaffle with the filling ingredients.

Nutrition: Calories: 186; Total Fat: 13.6g

Saturated Fat: 6.8g; **Cholesterol:** 120mg; **Sodium:** 342mg;

Total Carbs: 1.3g; **Fiber:** 0.4g; **Sugar**: 0.5g; **Protein**: 13.6g

24. Chocolate Oreo Sandwich Chaffles

✗ **Servings**: 2

🥄 **Preparation Time**: 0 Minutes

⏰ **Cooking Time**: 5 Minutes

📋 Ingredients :

For the Chaffles:

- ❖ 1 Organic egg
- ❖ 1 tablespoon heavy cream
- ❖ 2 tablespoons Erythritol
- ❖ 1½ tablespoons cacao powder
- ❖ 1 teaspoon coconut flour
- ❖ 2 tablespoons Erythritol
- ❖ ½ teaspoon organic baking powder
- ❖ ½ teaspoon organic vanilla extract

For the Filling:

- ❖ 3 tablespoons mascarpone cheese, softened

- ❖ 2 tablespoons heavy whipping cream
- ❖ ½ teaspoon organic vanilla extract
- ❖ 2 tablespoons powdered Erythritol

Directions:

1. Preheat a mini waffle maker and then grease it.

2. For the chaffles, in a medium bowl, put all ingredients and with a fork, mix until well combined.

3. Place half of the mixture into the preheated waffle iron and cook for about 3-5 minutes.

4. Repeat with the remaining mixture.

5. Meanwhile, for the filling, in a bowl, add all ingredients and mix well.

6. Spread the filling mixture over one chaffle and top with the remaining chaffle.

7. Cut in half and serve.

Nutrition: Calories: 168; Net Carbs: 3.2g; Fat: 14.4g;

Carbohydrates: 5g; Dietary Fiber:1.7g; Sugar: 0.4g;

Protein: 6.8g

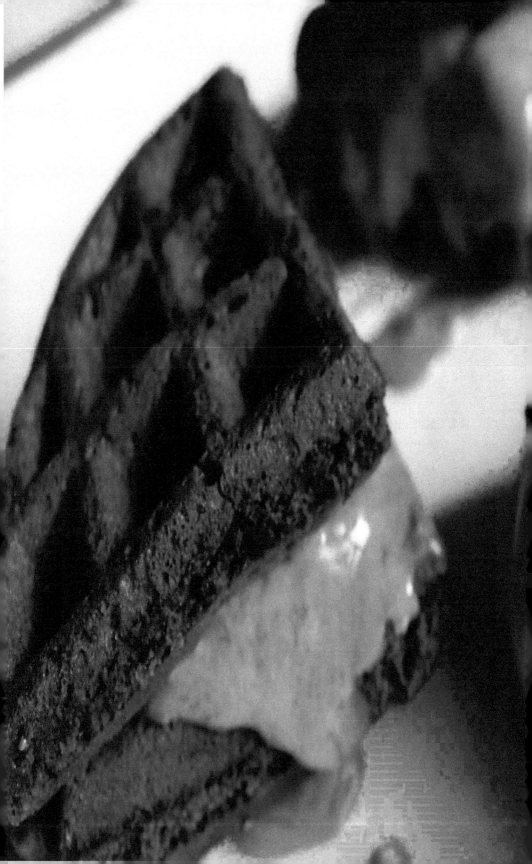

25. Peanut Butter Sandwich Chaffles

🍴 **Servings**: 2

🥄 **Preparation Time**: 10 Minutes

⏰ **Cooking Time**: 10 Minutes

📋 Ingredients :

For the Chaffles:

- ❖ 1 Organic egg, beaten

- ❖ 2 tablespoons almond flour

- ❖ ½ teaspoon organic baking powder

- ❖ ½ cup Mozzarella cheese, shredded

For the Filling:

- ❖ 2 tablespoons natural peanut butter

- ❖ 2 tablespoons heavy cream

- ❖ 2 teaspoons powdered Erythritol

Directions:

1. Preheat a mini waffle maker and then grease it.

2. For the chaffles, in a medium bowl, add all ingredients, and with a fork, mix until well combined.

3. Place half of the mixture into the preheated waffle iron and cook for about 3-5 minutes.

4. Repeat with the remaining mixture.

5. Meanwhile, for the filling, in a bowl, add all ingredients and mix well.

6. Spread the peanut butter mixture over one chaffle and top with the remaining chaffle.

7. Cut in half and serve.

Nutrition: Calories: 243; **Net Carbs**: 4.1g; **Fat**: 20.8g;

Carbohydrates: 5.8g; **Dietary Fiber**: 1.7g; **Sugar**: 1.9g;

Protein: 9.1g

26. Raisin Belgian Bread

X **Servings**: 2

✎ **Preparation Time**: 10 Minutes

⏰ **Cooking Time**: 10 Minutes

📋 Ingredients :

- ❖ 1 cup almond flour
- ❖ 1 tablespoon baking powder and caraway seeds
- ❖ 1 cup of butter and almond milk
- ❖ 1 tablespoon Raisins, honey, sugar-free maple syrup, and oil
- ❖ 1 teaspoon baking powder and cinnamon
- ❖ 2 eggs

Directions:

1. Take one bowl and add almond flour to it. Stir it with few seeds, baking powder.

2. Add salt, cinnamon, and raisins to it. Take another bowl, add almond milk and eggs to it.

3. Put some butter and honey in it. Place it into the flour mix.

4. Pour the mixture into the maker and cook it for 4 minutes.

5. Serve it with sugar-free maple syrup.

Nutrition: Calories: 1291; **Carbohydrates**: 60g;

Protein: 34g; **Fats:** 79g; **Saturated Fat**: 12.4g; **Fiber**: 30g;

Sugar: 11g

27. Keto Chocolate Chip Chaffle

X **Servings**: 1

🥄 **Preparation Time**: 5 Minutes

⏰ **Cooking Time**: 8 Minutes

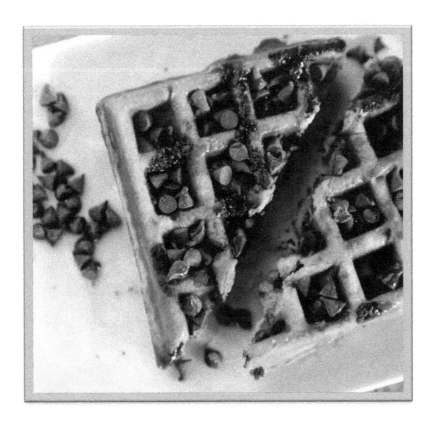

📋 **Ingredients :**

- ❖ 1 egg
- ❖ 1/4 teaspoon baking powder
- ❖ A pinch of salt
- ❖ 1 tablespoon heavy whipping cream (topping)
- ❖ 1/2 teaspoon coconut flour
- ❖ 1 tablespoon Chocolate Chips
- ❖ 1 cup mozzarella cheese

Directions:

1. Preheat the mini waffle maker until hot.

2. Whisk the egg in a bowl, add the cheese, and then mix well.

3. Stir in the remaining ingredients (except toppings, if any).

4. Grease the preheated waffle maker. This will help to create a crisper crust.

5. Scoop 1/2 of the batter onto the waffle maker, spread across evenly.

6. Sprinkle chocolate chips on top.

7. Cook until a bit browned and crispy, about 4 minutes.

8. Gently remove from the waffle maker and let it cool.

9. Repeat with the remaining batter.

10. Top with whipping cream.

11. Serve and Enjoy!

Nutrition: Calories: 110; **Carbs**: 16g; **Protein:** 6g;

Fats: 4g; **Phosphorus**: 138mg; **Potassium**: 745mg;

Sodium: 214mg

28.   Chocolate Chip Cannoli Chaffles

✗ **Servings**: 2

🥄 **Preparation Time**: 15 Minutes

⏰ **Cooking Time**: 5 Minutes

📋 Ingredients :

For the Chocolate Chip Chaffle:

- ❖ 1 tablespoon. butter, melted

- ❖ 1 tablespoon. monk fruit

- ❖ 1 egg yolk

- ❖ 1/8 teaspoon vanilla extract

- ❖ 3 tablespoon. almond flour

- ❖ 1/8 teaspoon baking powder

- ❖ 1 tablespoon. chocolate chips, sugar-free

For the Cannoli Topping:

- ❖ 2 oz. cream cheese
- ❖ 2 tablespoon. low-carb confectioners' sweetener
- ❖ 6 tablespoon. ricotta cheese, full fat
- ❖ 1/4 teaspoon vanilla extract
- ❖ 5 Drops lemon extract

Directions:

1. Preheat the mini waffle maker.

2. Mix all the ingredients for the chocolate chip chaffle in a mixing bowl. Combine well to make a batter.

3. Place half the batter on the waffle maker. Allow to cooking for 3-4 minutes.

4. While waiting for the chaffles to cooking, start making your cannoli topping by combining all ingredients until the consistency is creamy and smooth.

5. Place the cannoli topping on the cooked chaffles before serving.

Nutrition: Calories: 123; **Carbs:** 16.5g; **Protein:** 2g; **Fats:** 6g; **Phosphorus**: 56mg; **Potassium**: 450mg; **Sodium**: 35mg

29.   Oreo Chaffle

✕ **Servings**: 2

🖊 **Preparation Time**: 10 Minutes

⏰ **Cooking Time**: 20 Minutes

📋 **Ingredients :**

❖ 2 teaspoons coconut flour

❖ 3 tablespoons cocoa, unsweetened

❖ 1 teaspoon baking powder

❖ 4 tablespoons swerve sweetener

❖ 1 teaspoon vanilla extract, unsweetened

❖ 2 tablespoons heavy cream

❖ 2 eggs, at room temperature

❖ 2 tablespoons whipped cream

Directions:

1. Take a non-stick waffle iron, plug it in, select the

medium or medium-high heat setting and let it preheat until ready to use; it could also be indicated with an indicator light changing its color.

2. Meanwhile, mix the batter and for this, take a large bowl, add flour in it along with other ingredients and mix with an electric mixer until smooth.

3. Use a ladle to pour a quarter of the prepared batter into the heated waffle iron in a spiral direction, starting from the edges, then shut the lid and cook for 5 minutes or more until solid and nicely browned; the cooked waffle will look like a cake.

4. When done, transfer chaffles to a plate with a silicone spatula and repeat with the remaining batter.

5. When done, prepare the Oreo sandwiches, and for this, spread 1 tablespoon of whipped cream on one side of two chaffles and then cover with the remaining chaffles.

6. Serve immediately.

Nutrition: Calories: 295.6; Fats: 18.7g; Carbs: 11g;

Fiber: 2.2g; **Potassium**: 140mg; **Sodium:** 6.8mg;

Phosphorous:58g; **Protein**: 20.7g

30. Keto Ice Cream Chaffle

Servings: 2

Preparation Time: 15 Minutes

Cooking Time: 30 Minutes

Ingredients :

- ❖ 1 egg
- ❖ 2 tablespoons Swerve/Monk fruit
- ❖ 1 tablespoon Baking powder
- ❖ 1 tablespoon Heavy whipping cream
- ❖ Keto ice cream, as desired

Directions:

1. Take a small bowl and whisk the egg and add all the ingredients.

2. Beat until the mixture becomes creamy.

3. Pour the mixture into the lower plate of the waffle

maker and spread it evenly to cover the plate properly.

4. Close the lid.

5. Cook for at least 4 minutes to get the desired crunch.

6. Remove the chaffle from the heat and keep it aside for a few minutes.

7. Make as many chaffles as your mixture and waffle maker allow.

8. Top with your favorite ice cream, and enjoy!

Nutrition: Calories: 88; **Fat:** 1g; **Carbohydrates**: 19g;

Phosphorus: 74mg; **Potassium**: 92mg; **Sodium:** 47mg;

Protein: 1g

31. Broccoli & Almond Flour Chaffles

✗ **Servings**: 2

🥄 **Preparation Time**: 6 Minutes

⏰ **Cooking Time**: 8 Minutes

📋 Ingredients :

- ❖ 1 Organic egg, beaten
- ❖ ½ cup Cheddar cheese, shredded
- ❖ ¼ cup fresh broccoli, chopped
- ❖ 1 tablespoon almond flour
- ❖ ¼ teaspoon garlic powder

Directions:

1. Preheat a mini waffle maker and then grease it.

2. In a bowl, place all ingredients and mix until well combined.

3. Place half of the mixture into the preheated waffle iron

and cook for about four minutes or until golden brown.

4. Repeat with the remaining mixture.

5. Serve warm.

Nutrition: Calories: 221; **Protein:** 17g **Carbs:** 31g;

Fat: 8g; **Sodium:** (Na) 235mg **Potassium:** (K) 176mg;

Phosphorus: 189mg

32. Cheddar Jalapeño Chaffle

X **Servings**: 2

🥄 **Preparation Time**: 6 Minutes

⏰ **Cooking Time**: 5 Minutes

📋 Ingredients :

- ❖ 2 large eggs

- ❖ ½ cup shredded mozzarella

- ❖ ¼ cup almond flour

- ❖ ½ teaspoon baking powder

- ❖ ¼ cup shredded cheddar cheese

- ❖ 2 tablespoons diced jalapeños jarred or canned

For the Toppings:

- ❖ ½ Cooked bacon, chopped

- ❖ 2 tablespoons cream cheese

❖ ¼ Jalapeño slices

Directions:

1. Turn on the waffle maker to heat and oil it with cooking spray.

2. Mix the mozzarella, eggs, baking powder, almond flour, and garlic powder in a bowl.

3. Sprinkle two tablespoons cheddar cheese in a thin layer on the waffle maker, and ½ jalapeño.

4. Ladle half of the egg mixture on top of the cheese and jalapeños.

5. Cook for 4-5 minutes, or until done.

6. Repeat for the second chaffle.

7. Top with cream cheese, bacon, and jalapeño slices.

Nutrition: Calories: 221; **Protein:** 13g; **Carbs:** 1g;

Fat: 34g; **Sodium:** (Na) 80mg; **Potassium:** (K) 119mg;

Phosphorus: 158mg

33. Taco Chaffles

Servings: 2

Preparation Time: 10 Minutes

Cooking Time: 20 Minutes

Ingredients :

- 1 tablespoon almond flour

- 1 cup taco blend cheese

- 2 organic eggs

- 1/4 teaspoon taco seasoning

Directions:

1. Preheat a mini waffle maker and then grease it.

2. In a bowl, place all ingredients and mix until well combined.

3. Place ¼ of the mixture into the preheated waffle iron and cook for about four minutes or until golden brown.

4. Repeat with the remaining mixture.

5. Serve warm.

Nutrition: **Calories:** 221; **Protein**: 14g; **Carbs**: 3g; **Fat**: 2g;

Sodium: (Na) 119mg; **Potassium**: (K) 398mg;

Phosphorus: 149mg

34. Spinach & Cauliflower Chaffles

✗ **Servings**: 2

🥄 **Preparation Time**: 6 Minutes

⏰ **Cooking Time**: 10 Minutes

📋 Ingredients :

❖ ½ cup frozen chopped spinach, thawed and squeezed

❖ ½ cup cauliflower, chopped finely

❖ ½ cup Cheddar cheese, shredded

❖ ½ cup Mozzarella cheese, shredded

❖ 1/3 cup Parmesan cheese, shredded

❖ 2 organic eggs

❖ 1 tablespoon butter, melted

❖ 1 teaspoon garlic powder

❖ 1 teaspoon onion powder

❖ Salt and freshly ground black pepper, to taste

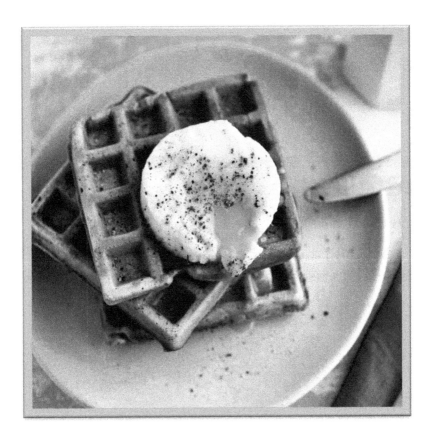

Directions:

1. Preheat a waffle iron and then grease it.

2. In a medium bowl, place all ingredients and mix until well combined.

3. Place half of the mixture into the preheated waffle iron

and cook for about 4-5 minutes or until golden brown.

4. Repeat with the remaining mixture.

5. Serve warm.

Nutrition: Calories: 221; **Protein**: 11g; **Carbs**: 26g;

Fat: 7g; **Sodium**: (Na) 143mg; **Potassium**: (K)197mg;

Phosphorus: 182mg

35. Rosemary in Chaffles

✖ **Servings**: 2

✎ **Preparation Time**: 6 Minutes

⏰ **Cooking Time**: 8 Minutes

🗒 Ingredients :

- ❖ 1 organic egg, beaten
- ❖ ½ cup Cheddar cheese, shredded
- ❖ 1 tablespoon almond flour
- ❖ 1 tablespoon fresh rosemary, chopped
- ❖ A pinch of salt and freshly ground black pepper

Directions:

1. Preheat a mini waffle maker and then grease it.

2. For the chaffles, in a medium bowl, place all ingredients and with a fork, mix until well combined.

3. Place half of the mixture into the preheated waffle iron and cook for about four minutes or until golden brown.

4. Repeat with the remaining mixture.

5. Serve warm.

Nutrition: Calories: 221; Protein: 12g; Carbs: 29g; Fat: 8g; Sodium: (Na) 398mg; Potassium: (K) 347mg; Phosphorus: 241mg

Blackberry Ricotta Chaffles

🍴 **Servings**: 2

🥄 **Preparation Time**: 5 Minutes

⏰ **Cooking Time**: 5 Minutes

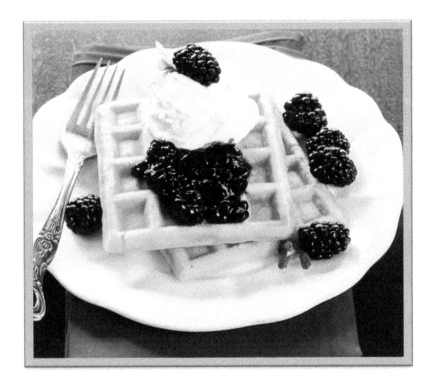

📋 **Ingredients :**

For the Chaffles:

- ❖ 2 Large organic eggs

- ❖ 1 cup Mozzarella cheese, shredded finely

For the Filling:

- ❖ ¼ cup fresh blackberries

- ❖ 4 teaspoons ricotta cheese, crumbled

Directions:

1. Preheat a mini waffle maker and then grease it.

2. For the chaffles, in a bowl, add the eggs and cheese and stir to combine.

3. Place ¼ of the mixture into the preheated waffle iron and cook for about 3-4 minutes.

4. Repeat with the remaining mixture.

5. Place the filling ingredients over two chaffles and top with remaining chaffles.

6. Cut each in half and serve.

Nutrition: Calories: 67; Net Carbs: 1.1g; Fat: 4.2g;

Carbohydrates: 1.6g; **Dietary Fiber**: 0.5g; **Sugar**: 0.7g;

Protein: 5.9g

36. Raspberry Sandwich Chaffles

✗ **Servings**: 2

🥄 **Preparation Time**: 15 Minutes

⏰ **Cooking Time**: 10 Minutes

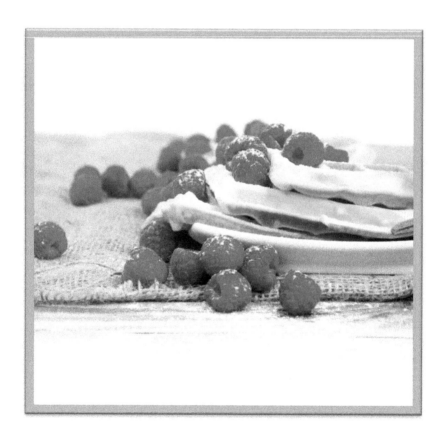

📋 Ingredients :

For the Chaffles:

- ❖ 1 Organic egg, beaten
- ❖ 1 teaspoon organic vanilla extract
- ❖ 1 tablespoon almond flour
- ❖ 1 teaspoon organic baking powder
- ❖ A pinch of ground cinnamon
- ❖ 1 cup Mozzarella cheese, shredded

For the Filling:

- ❖ 2 tablespoons cream cheese, softened
- ❖ 2 tablespoons Erythritol
- ❖ ¼ teaspoon organic vanilla extract
- ❖ 4 Fresh raspberries, chopped

Directions:

1. Preheat a mini waffle maker and then grease it.

2. For the chaffles, in a bowl, add the egg and vanilla extract and mix well.

3. Add the flour, baking powder, and cinnamon and mix until well combined.

4. Add the Mozzarella cheese and stir to combine.

5. Place half of the mixture into the preheated waffle iron and cook for about 4-5 minutes.

6. Repeat with the remaining mixture.

7. Meanwhile, for the filling, in a bowl, place all the ingredients except the strawberry pieces, and with a hand mixer, beat until well combined.

8. Spread cream cheese mixture over one chaffle and top with raspberries.

9. Cover with remaining chaffle.

10. Cut in half and serve.

Nutrition: Calories: 143; **Net Carbs**: 6.6g; **Fat**: 10.1g;

Carbohydrates: 4.1g; **Dietary Fiber**: 0.8g; **Sugar**: 1.2g;

Protein: 0.8g

37.   Berries Sauce Sandwich Chaffles

X **Servings**: 2

✎ **Preparation Time**: 10 Minutes

⏰ **Cooking Time**: 8 Minutes

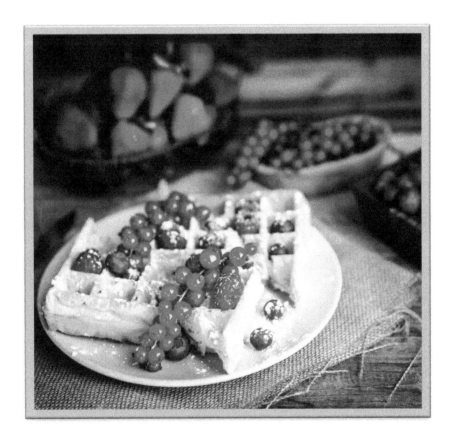

📋 **Ingredients :**

For the Filling:

- ❖ 3 Ounces frozen mixed berries, thawed with the juice
- ❖ 1 tablespoon Erythritol
- ❖ 1 tablespoon water
- ❖ ¼ tablespoon fresh lemon juice
- ❖ 2 teaspoons cream

For the Chaffles:

- ❖ 1 Large organic egg, beaten
- ❖ ½ cup Cheddar cheese, shredded
- ❖ 2 tablespoons almond flour

Directions:

1. For the berry sauce, in a pan, add the berries, Erythritol, water, and lemon juice over medium heat and cook for about 8-10 minutes, pressing with the spoon occasionally.

2. Remove the pan of sauce from the heat and set it aside to cool before serving.

3. Preheat a mini waffle maker and then grease it.

4. In a bowl, add the egg, Cheddar cheese, and almond flour and beat until well combined.

5. Place half of the mixture into the preheated waffle iron and cook for about 3-5 minutes.

6. Repeat with the remaining mixture.

7. Spread berry sauce over one chaffle and top with the remaining chaffle.

8. Cut in half and serve.

Nutrition: Calories: 222; Net Carbs: 4.7g; Fat: 21.5g; Carbohydrates: 7g; Dietary Fiber: 2.3g; Sugar: 3.8g; Protein: 10.5g

38. Grilled Cheese Sandwich Chaffles

✗ **Servings**: 2

🥄 **Preparation Time**: 5 Minutes

⏰ **Cooking Time**: 5 Minutes

📋 **Ingredients :**

For the Chaffles:

- ❖ 1 Organic egg
- ❖ ½ cup Cheddar cheese, shredded
- ❖ ¼ teaspoon garlic powder

For the Filling:

- ❖ 1 tablespoon butter
- ❖ ¼ cup Cheddar cheese, shredded

Directions:

1. Preheat a mini waffle maker and then grease it.

2. In a bowl, add the egg, Cheddar cheese, and almond flour and beat until well combined.

3. Place half of the mixture into the preheated waffle iron and cook for about 3-4 minutes.

4. Repeat with the remaining mixture.

5. In a frying pan, melt the butter over medium heat.

6. Cover with the second chaffle and cook for about 1 minute per side.

7. Transfer the chaffle sandwich onto a plate and cut it in half.

8. Serve immediately.

Nutrition: Calories: 254; **Net Carbs**: 1g; **Fat**: 22g;

Carbohydrates: 1g; **Dietary Fiber**: 0g; **Sugar**: 0.5g;

Protein: 13.4g

39. Mozzarella Lemony Chaffles

🍴 **Servings**: 2

🥄 **Preparation Time**: 5 Minutes

⏰ **Cooking Time**: 17 Minutes

📋 Ingredients :

- ❖ 2 eggs
- ❖ 1 cup Shredded mozzarella
- ❖ 2 tablespoons Lemon juice
- ❖ 2 teaspoons Any keto sweetener
- ❖ 2 teaspoons Coconut flour

Directions:

1. Preheat your mini waffle iron if needed and grease it.

2. Mix all the ingredients in a bowl and whisk.

3. Cook your mixture in the mini waffle iron for at least 4 minutes.

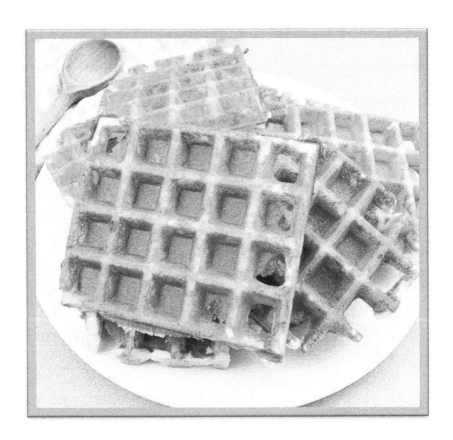

4. Serve hot and make as many chaffles as your mixture and waffle maker allow.

40.   Double Chocolate Chaffle

X **Servings**: 2

Preparation Time: 5 Minutes

Cooking Time: 10 Minutes

📋 Ingredients :

- ❖ 2 eggs
- ❖ 4 tablespoons Coconut flour
- ❖ 2 tablespoons Cocoa powder
- ❖ 2 oz. Cream cheese
- ❖ ½ teaspoon Baking powder
- ❖ 2 tablespoons (unsweetened) Chocolate chips
- ❖ 1 teaspoon Vanilla extract
- ❖ 4 tablespoons Swerve/Monk fruit

Directions:

1. Preheat a mini waffle maker if needed and grease it.

2. In a mixing bowl, beat the eggs.

3. In a separate mixing bowl, add coconut flour, cocoa powder, Swerve/Monk fruit, and baking powder; when combined, pour into the eggs with cream cheese and vanilla extracts.

4. Mix them all well to give them uniform consistency, and pour the mixture to the lower plate of the waffle maker.

5. On top of the mixture, sprinkle a half teaspoon of unsweetened chocolate chips around and close the lid.

6. Cook for at least 4 minutes to get the desired crunch.

7. Remove the chaffle from the heat and keep it aside for around one minute.

8. Make as many chaffles as your mixture and waffle maker allow.

9. Serve with your favorite whipped cream or berries.

Nutrition: Calories: 87; Fat: 1g; Carbohydrates: 22g;

Phosphorus: 28mg; Potassium: 192mg; Sodium: 3mg;

Protein: 1g

41. Cream Cheese Mini Chaffle

✗ **Servings**: 2

🖋 **Preparation Time**: 5 Minutes

⏰ **Cooking Time**: 10 Minutes

📋 Ingredients :

- ❖ 1 egg
- ❖ 2 tablespoons Coconut flour
- ❖ 1 oz. Cream cheese
- ❖ 1/4 teaspoon Baking powder
- ❖ 1/2 teaspoon Vanilla extract
- ❖ 4 teaspoons Swerve/Monk fruit

Directions:

1. Preheat a waffle maker and grease it if needed.

2. In a mixing bowl, mix coconut flour, Swerve/Monk fruit, and baking powder.

3. Now add the egg to the mixture with cream cheese and vanilla extract.

4. Mix them all well and pour the mixture to the lower plate of the waffle maker.

5. Close the lid.

6. Cook for at least 4 minutes to get the desired crunch.

7. Remove the chaffle from the heat.

8. Make as many chaffles as your mixture and waffle maker allow.

9. Eat the chaffles with your favorite toppings.

Nutrition: Calories: 47; Fat: 0g; Carbohydrates: 11g;

Phosphorus: 30mg; **Potassium:** 197mg; **Sodium:** 4mg;

Protein: 1g

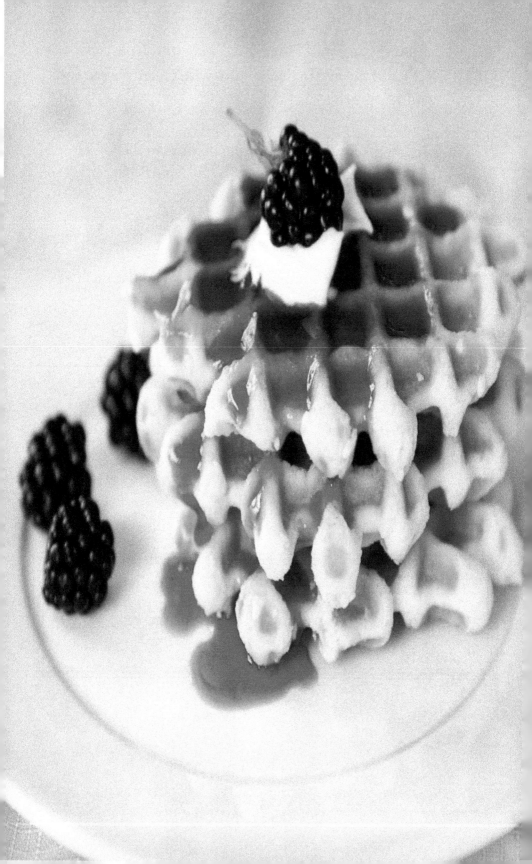

42. Blackberries Chaffle

✖ Servings: 2

✒ Preparation Time: 15 Minutes

⏰ Cooking Time: 20 Minutes

📋 Ingredients :

- ❖ 1/3 cup Cheddar cheese
- ❖ 1 egg
- ❖ 1/2 cup Blackberries
- ❖ 2 tablespoons Almond flour
- ❖ 1/4 teaspoon Baking powder
- ❖ 2 tablespoons ground almonds
- ❖ 1/3 cup mozzarella cheese

Directions:

1. Mix cheddar cheese, egg, blackberries, almond flour, almond ground, and baking powder together in a bowl.

2. Preheat your waffle iron and grease it.

3. In your mini waffle iron, shred half of the Mozzarella

cheese.

4. Add the mixture to your mini waffle iron.

5. Again, shred the remaining mozzarella cheese on the mixture.

6. Cook till the desired crisp is achieved.

7. Make as many chaffles as your mixture and waffle maker allow.

Nutrition: Calories: 243; Fat: 11g; Carbohydrates: 33g; Phosphorus: 84mg; **Potassium**: 189mg; **Sodium**: 145mg; Protein: 4g

43. Bacon, egg & Avocado Chaffle Sandwich

🍴 **Servings**: 2

🥄 **Preparation Time**: 10 Minutes

⏰ **Cooking Time**: 10 Minutes

📋 Ingredients :

❖ Cooking spray

❖ 4 Bacon Slices

❖ 2 eggs

❖ ½ Avocado, mashed

❖ 4 Basic chaffles

❖ 2 Lettuce leaves

Directions:

1. Coat your skillet with cooking spray.

2. Cook the bacon until golden and crisp.

3. Transfer into a paper towel-lined plate.

4. Break the eggs into the same pan and cook until firm.

5. Flip and cook until the yolk is set.

6. Spread the avocado on the chaffle.

7. Top with lettuce, egg, and bacon.

8. Top with another chaffle.

Nutrition: Calories: 372; Total Fat: 30.1g; Saturated Fat: 8.6g; **Cholesterol:** 205mg; **Sodium:** 3mg; **Total Carbohydrates**: 5.4g; **Dietary Fiber**: 3.4g; **Total Sugars**: 0.6g **Protein**: 20.6g; **Potassium**: 524mg

44. Breakfast Spinach Ricotta Chaffles

🍴 **Servings**: 2

🥄 **Preparation Time**: 8 Minutes

⏰ **Cooking Time**: 28 Minutes

📋 Ingredients :

- ❖ 4 oz. Frozen spinach, thawed, squeezed dry

- ❖ 1 cup ricotta cheese
- ❖ 2 eggs, beaten
- ❖ ½ teaspoon garlic powder
- ❖ ¼ cup finely grated Pecorino Romano cheese
- ❖ ½ cup finely grated mozzarella cheese
- ❖ Salt
- ❖ Freshly ground black pepper to taste

Directions:

1. Preheat the waffle iron.

2. In a bowl, add all ingredients.

3. Open the iron, lightly grease with cooking spray, and spoon in a quarter of the mixture.

4. Close the iron and cook until brown and crispy, 7 minutes.

5. Remove the chaffle onto a plate and set it aside.

6. Make three more chaffles with the remaining mixture.

7. Allow cooling and serve afterward.

Nutrition: Calories: 1; **Fats**: 13.15g; **Carbs**: 5.06g; **Net Carbs**: 4.06g; **Protein**: 12.79g

45. Pumpkin Chaffle With Frosting

X **Servings**: 2

✎ **Preparation Time**: 10 Minutes

⏰ **Cooking Time**: 15 Minutes

📋 Ingredients :

- ❖ 1 egg, lightly beaten
- ❖ 1 tablespoon sugar-free pumpkin puree
- ❖ 1/4 teaspoon pumpkin pie spice
- ❖ 1/2 cup mozzarella cheese, shredded

For the frosting:

- ❖ 1/2 teaspoon vanilla
- ❖ 2 tablespoons Swerve
- ❖ 2 tablespoons cream cheese, softened

Directions:

1. Preheat your waffle maker.

2. Add the egg to a bowl and whisk well.

3. Add pumpkin puree, pumpkin pie spice, and cheese and stir well.

4. Spray the waffle maker with cooking spray.

5. Pour 1/2 of the batter in the hot waffle maker and cook for 3-4 minutes or until golden brown. Repeat with the remaining batter.

6. In a small bowl, mix all frosting ingredients until smooth.

7. Add frosting on top of hot chaffles and serve.

Nutrition: Calories: 9.7; Carbohydrates: 3.6; Sugar: 0.6;

Protein: 5.6; Cholesterol: 97mg

46. Chaffle Strawberry Sandwich

✗ **Servings**: 2

🥄 **Preparation Time**: 7 Minutes

⏲ **Cooking Time**: 5 Minutes

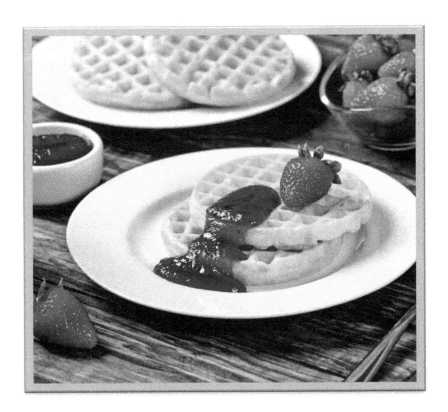

▤ **Ingredients :**

- ❖ 1/4 cup heavy cream
- ❖ 4 oz. Strawberry slice

Chaffle Ingredients:

- ❖ 1 egg
- ❖ ½ cup mozzarella cheese

Directions:

1. Make two chaffles with the mentioned ingredients.

2. Meanwhile, mix cream and strawberries.

3. Spread this mixture over a chaffle slice.

4. Drizzle chocolate sauce over a sandwich.

5. Serve and enjoy!

Nutrition: Protein:4; Fat:196; Carbohydrates: 10

47. New Year Keto Chaffle Cake

X **Servings**: 2

🥄 **Preparation Time**: 0 Minutes

⏰ **Cooking Time**: 15 Minutes

📋 Ingredients :

- ❖ 4 oz. Almond flour
- ❖ 2 cup cheddar cheese
- ❖ 5 eggs
- ❖ 1 teaspoon stevia
- ❖ 2 teaspoons baking powder
- ❖ 2 teaspoons vanilla extract
- ❖ 1/4 cup almond butter, melted
- ❖ 3 tablespoons Almond milk
- ❖ 1 cup cranberries
- ❖ I cup coconut cream

Directions:

1. Break the eggs into a small mixing bowl, mix the eggs, almond flour, Stevia, and baking powder.

2. Add the melted butter slowly to the flour mixture, mix well to ensure a smooth consistency.

3. Add the cheese, almond milk, cranberries, and vanilla to the flour and butter mixture; be sure to mix well.

4. Preheat the waffles maker and grease it with avocado oil.

5. Pour some mixture into the waffle maker and cook until golden brown.

6. Make five chaffles

7. Stag chaffles on a plate. Spread the cream all around.

8. Cut in slice and serve.

Nutrition: Protein:15; Fat:207; Carbohydrates: 15

48. Walnut Pumpkin Chaffles

X **Servings**: 2

🖊 **Preparation Time**: 10 Minutes

⏰ **Cooking Time**: 10 Minutes

📋 Ingredients :

- ❖ 1 Organic egg, beaten
- ❖ ½ cup Mozzarella cheese, shredded
- ❖ 2 tablespoons almond flour
- ❖ 1 tablespoon sugar-free pumpkin puree
- ❖ 1 teaspoon Erythritol
- ❖ ¼ teaspoon ground cinnamon
- ❖ 2 tablespoons walnuts, toasted and chopped

Directions:

1. Preheat a mini waffle maker and then grease it.

2. In a bowl, place all ingredients except walnuts and beat

until well combined.

3. Fold in the walnuts.

4. Place half of the mixture into the preheated waffle iron and cook for about 5 minutes or until golden brown.

5. Repeat with the remaining mixture.

6. Serve warm.

Nutrition: Calories: 148; **Net Carbs**: 1.6g **Fat**: 11.8g;

Saturated Fat: 2g; **Carbohydrates**: 3.3g; **Dietary Fiber**: 1.7g;

Sugar: 0.8g; **Protein**:6.7g

---

49. Pumpkin Cream Cheese Chaffles

✖ **Servings**: 2

🥄 **Preparation Time**: 10 Minutes

⏰ **Cooking Time**: 10 Minutes

📋 Ingredients :

- ❖ 1 Organic egg, beaten
- ❖ ½ cup Mozzarella cheese, shredded
- ❖ 1½ tablespoon sugar-free pumpkin puree
- ❖ 2 teaspoons heavy cream
- ❖ 1 teaspoon cream cheese, softened
- ❖ 1 tablespoon almond flour
- ❖ 1 tablespoon Erythritol
- ❖ ½ teaspoon pumpkin pie spice
- ❖ ½ teaspoon organic baking powder
- ❖ 1 teaspoon organic vanilla extract

Directions:

1. Preheat a mini waffle maker and then grease it.

2. In a medium bowl, place all ingredients, and with a fork, mix until well combined.

3. Place half of the mixture into the preheated waffle iron and cook for about 3-5 minutes or until golden brown.

4. Repeat with the remaining mixture.

5. Serve warm.

Nutrition: Calories: 110; NetCarbs:2.5g; Fat: 4.3g;

Saturated Fat: 1g; **Carbohydrates:** 3.3g; **Dietary Fiber:** 0.8g;

Sugar: 1g; **Protein:** 5.2g

50. Whipping Cream Pumpkin Chaffles

✗ **Servings**: 2

✎ **Preparation Time**: 10 Minutes

⏰ **Cooking Time**: 12 Minutes

📋 Ingredients :

- ❖ 2 Organic eggs
- ❖ 2 tablespoons homemade pumpkin puree
- ❖ 2 tablespoons heavy whipping cream
- ❖ 1 tablespoon coconut flour
- ❖ 1 tablespoon Erythritol
- ❖ 1 teaspoon pumpkin pie spice
- ❖ ½ teaspoon organic baking powder
- ❖ ½ teaspoon organic vanilla extract
- ❖ A pinch of salt
- ❖ ½ cup Mozzarella cheese, shredded

Directions:

1. Preheat a mini waffle maker and then grease it.

2. In a bowl, place all the ingredients except Mozzarella cheese and beat until well combined.

3. Add the Mozzarella cheese and stir to combine.

4. Place half of the mixture into the preheated waffle iron and cook for about 4-6 minutes or until golden brown.

5. Repeat with the remaining mixture.

6. Serve warm.

Nutrition: Calories: 81; Net Carbs: 2.1g; Fat: 5.9g;

Saturated Fat: 3g; Carbohydrates: 3.1g; Dietary Fiber: 1g;

Sugar: 0.5g; Protein:4.3g

51. Chocolate Cream Chaffles

🍴 **Servings**: 2

🥄 **Preparation Time**: 10 Minutes

⏰ **Cooking Time**: 10 Minutes

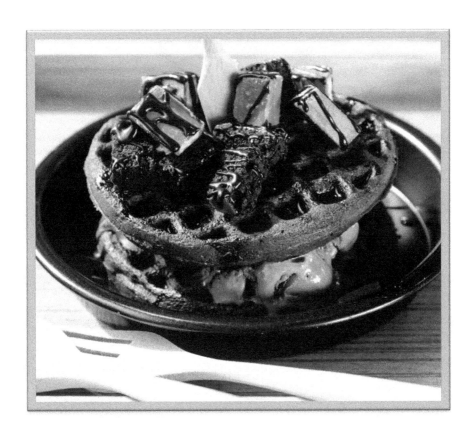

📋 Ingredients :

- ❖ 1 Organic egg
- ❖ 1½ tablespoons cacao powder
- ❖ 2 tablespoons Erythritol
- ❖ 1 tablespoon heavy cream
- ❖ 1 teaspoon coconut flour
- ❖ ½ teaspoon organic baking powder
- ❖ ½ teaspoon organic vanilla extract
- ❖ ½ teaspoon powdered Erythritol

Directions:

1. Preheat a mini waffle maker and then grease it.

2. In a bowl, place all ingredients except the powdered Erythritol and beat until well combined.

3. Place half of the mixture into the preheated waffle iron and cook for about 3-5 minutes or until golden brown.

4. Repeat with the remaining mixture.

5. Serve warm with the sprinkling of powdered Erythritol.

Nutrition: Calories: 76; Net Carbs: 2.1g; Fat: 5.9g

Saturated Fat: 3g; Carbohydrates: 3.8g

Dietary Fiber: 1.7g; Sugar: 0.3g; Protein: 3.8g

CONCLUSION

The diet increases immunity; if you have immunity issues, the best way to boost it is to switch to foods that will reduce the risk for you to catch common colds, flu, and other inflammations. Everybody needs a strong immune system. If this diet showed a gradual improvement of the immune system in cancer patients only after one month, you could only imagine how well a healthy person will react to keto foods.

It increases a good mental state. Autistic and bipolar patients are often advised to eat keto meals. Many studies show that treating autistic children with the Ketogenic diet for six months showed improvement in their mental and behavioral state. Keeping patients with autism or any other mental disorder in a good mental state needs is crucial.

The keto diet is a perfect way to keep you in a stable mood and will not cause you mood swings (which unfortunately often happens when you eat food rich in carbs).

Talking about Epilepsy, the Ketogenic diet was primarily developed to treat epileptic children with frequent seizures. About one century ago, when keto was first discovered, it significantly reduced epileptic seizures in children, ever since it is recommended for patients with epilepsy.

It is good for your general health. Your diet can either kill you or cure you. It does not matter why you start following the keto diet (weight loss, immunity system, energy, strength, etc.); it will improve your general health for the better.

The keto meals are delicious enough, so that can be a good reason to start following it even if you don't need to lose weight. You will let go of your old eating habits, become more aware of what you eat, and your energy levels will rise.

The keto diet will provide you with the most important nutrients, healthy fats, proteins, and fiber, healthy oils (coconut, avocado, and olive).

You will see that there are many healthy and great food substitutes for all the unhealthy and junk food you used to eat. As the ketones in your body rise, your immune system will be put in balance, your skin, hair, and nails will become stronger, and you will keep your cholesterol and triglycerides under control.

Finally, one of the biggest reasons to start following this diet is the fact that there are no side effects; keto meals cannot harm you at all. The biggest challenge will last for a few days when you will quit eating carbohydrates (bread, pasta, sweets), but once you get used to the new foods, you will not even think twice about going back.

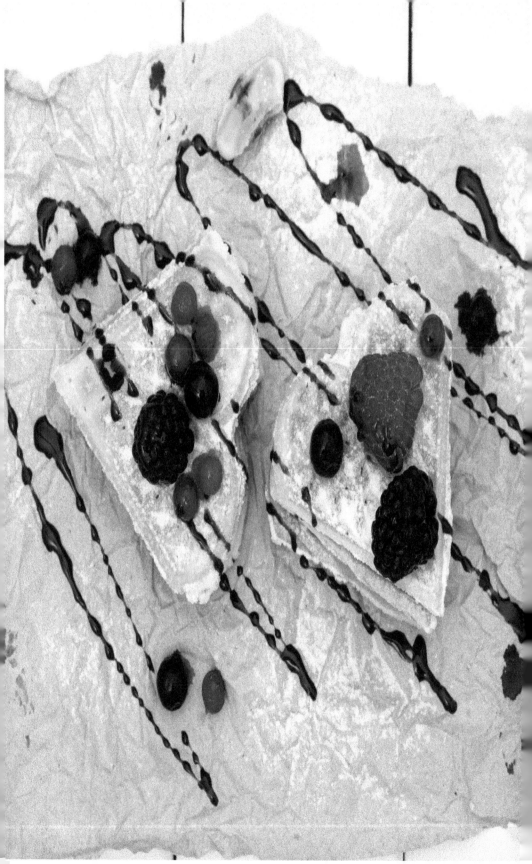

Lightning Source UK Ltd.
Milton Keynes UK
UKHW020747250621
386136UK00005B/27